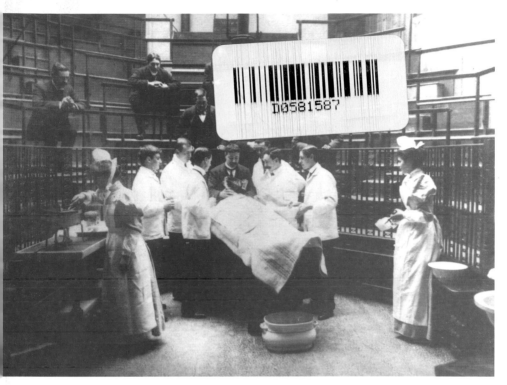

An operation in progress at University College Medical School, London. Before the acceptance of the germ theory, the operating theatre was the dirtiest room in the hospital. By 1898, when this picture was taken, the doctors wore white coats, but not masks or gloves. Students observed the operation from the amphitheatre wearing their ordinary clothes.

The Victorian Hospital

Lavinia Mitton

A Shire book

Contents

ACKNOWLEDGEMENTS

Many people gave advice and assistance in the preparation of this book. I wish particularly to thank Eleanor James, Judy Slinn, and Jacqueline and Simon Mitton. Illustrations are acknowledged as follows: the Florence Nightingale Museum, page 5 (centre); The Old Operating Theatre, Museum and Herb Garrett, page 8 (top); the Science and Society Picture Library, page 1; the Amoret Tanner Collection, pages 15 (top and centre), 28 (bottom). The photographs on pages 17 (bottom two), 19 (bottom), 20, 24 (top), 27 (bottom), 29 and 30 are by the author.

Cover: 'The Old Operating Theatre at the London Hospital Demolished in 1889', an oil painting by F. M. Harvey. (Copyright: The Royal London Hospital Archives and Museum)

British Library Cataloguing in Publication Data: Mitton, Lavinia. The Victorian hospital. – (Shire album; 356). 1. Hospital care – Great Britain – History – 19th century. 2. Hospitals – Great Britain – History – 19th century. I. Title. 326.1'1'0941'09034 ISBN 0 7478 0487 7.

Published in 2004 by Shire Publications Ltd, Cromwell House, Church Street, Princes Risborough, Buckinghamshire HP27 9AA, UK. (Website: www.shirebooks.co.uk)

Copyright © 2001 by Lavinia Mitton. First published 2001; reprinted 2004. Shire Album 356. ISBN 0 7478 0487 7. Lavinia Mitton is hereby identified as the author of this work in accordance with Section 77 of the Copyright, Designs and Patents Act 1988.

Printed in Great Britain by CIT Printing Services Ltd, Press Buildings, Merlins Bridge, Haverfordwest, Pembrokeshire SA61 1XF.

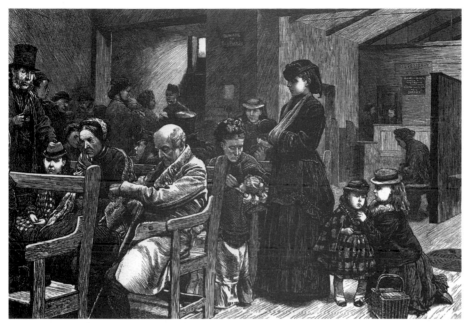

The out-patients' department at University College Hospital, London. The number of people applying for treatment as out-patients at general hospitals rose steadily in the first half of the nineteenth century. Victorian hospitals usually had extensive out-patient departments. In 1870 10,000 casualties and 18,000 out-patients were seen at University College Hospital. The development of out-patient departments was not welcomed by GPs, who feared the competition. (Engraving from 'The Graphic', 6th January 1872.)

Victorian hospitals and medical advances

Overcrowding in the wards, surgery without anaesthesia, and the danger of catching a deadly infection: this was the experience of a sick person in hospital in the 1830s. It is difficult to imagine how the patient must have felt as he lay upon the wooden operating table, eyes to the rafters, listening for the surgeon's footstep that signalled the terrible moment was nigh!

In Victorian times the wealthy paid a doctor to attend them at home and the poor had to turn to a charitable hospital or, worse, the dreaded workhouse infirmary. Victorian hospitals were run either as charities or by the local authorities. The philanthropic voluntary hospital movement first arose in the eighteenth century when there were only a handful of hospitals in the whole of Britain. The number increased rapidly in the nineteenth century. Not all kinds of cases were admitted to the voluntary, mainly 'general', hospitals: children, incurables, patients with chronic or infectious diseases, the mentally ill and pregnant women were usually excluded, so specialist institutions were set up to fill the gaps left by the voluntary system. Local authorities ran pauper workhouse infirmaries, isolation hospitals and the county lunatic asylums. The way the hospital was run, the design of its buildings and the quality of care provided varied according to the type of hospital.

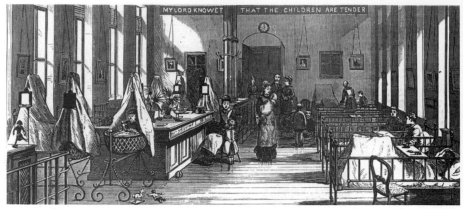

A ward at the East London Hospital for Children. One of the first children's hospitals was Great Ormond Street in London, founded in 1852. By 1888 there were thirty-eight children's hospitals in Britain. Children's hospitals concentrated on acute cases or those needing urgent treatment. Children with chronic bone and joint disease were treated in separate institutions. However, under the National Health Service, it was believed that children were best cared for within a general hospital. (Engraving from 'The Graphic', 21st December 1878.)

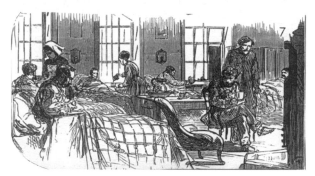

A ward scene at the Charing Cross Hospital, London. Such voluntary hospitals were predominantly for poorer patients, from whom gratitude and deference to their superiors were expected. The patients' day was organised for the convenience of the staff, with waking hours very early, and visits were restricted. In teaching hospitals, belittling patients as simply a 'case' for the education of students had the effect of degrading them even more. (Engraving from 'The Graphic', 31st March 1877.)

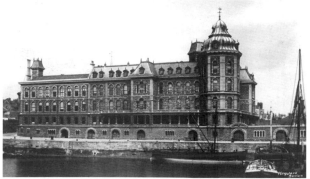

A postcard of Bristol General Hospital, established in 1832. Most general voluntary hospitals were founded in England and Wales between 1730 and 1850. By 1861 there were 230 voluntary hospitals, with 14,800 beds. This new building was erected in 1856–7 and included an out-patient department big enough to accommodate over 300 patients. The basement was designed as warehousing for the nearby harbour, thus providing an income for the hospital.

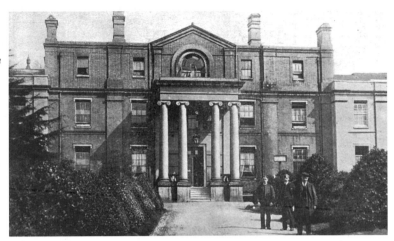

East Suffolk Hospital, Ipswich, founded in 1835 as a voluntary hospital and closed in the mid 1980s. As towns grew during the Industrial Revolution, hospitals were established in most urban areas. They were a source of civic pride along with the town hall and public library.

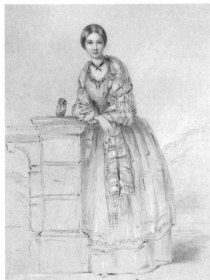

There was great potential for the spread of disease within the hospital environment before the mid nineteenth century. Early Victorians believed that disease was caused by foul air, or miasma, given off by stagnant water and stinking cesspools. It was thought that after a certain time the walls, ceilings and floors of hospitals became saturated with 'mephitic odours' which were a source of infection. Reducing the intake of these noxious vapours would reduce the likelihood of catching a disease. By the 1850s this idea was being challenged by the theory that disease was spread by germs. However, the influential hospital reformer Florence Nightingale was a staunch miasmatist, and the design of hospital wards constructed in the late-Victorian period reflects her ideas and her ambition 'to do the sick no harm'.

Above: *Lithograph of Florence Nightingale with Athena the Owl after a drawing by Parthenope Nightingale. Historians no longer credit Florence Nightingale exclusively with the rise of modern nursing. Her ideas for reform based on training and discipline were already around at the time she went to the Crimea. Nevertheless, to the public, the 'Lady with the Lamp' was a heroine. The Nightingale Fund Training School for Nurses at St Thomas's Hospital was established with money given by the public in her honour.*

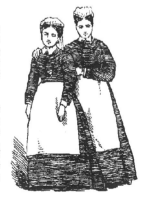

Right: *Nursing changed enormously during Queen Victoria's reign. Before the nurse training schools were set up under Florence Nightingale's influence nursing was not a respectable occupation. She commented that nursing was generally done by those 'who were too old, too weak, too drunken, too dirty, too stolid, or too bad to do anything else'. Nursing was an unskilled job and nurses spent much of their time cooking and scrubbing. No doubt the conditions before reform have been exaggerated but it is not surprising that the poor had a horror of hospitals. (Illustration from 'The Hospital', 19th June 1897.)*

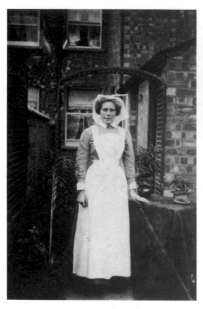

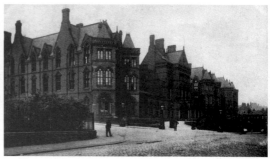

Above: *A postcard of Leeds Infirmary. Founded in 1767 as a voluntary hospital, a new Gothic-style infirmary was built to replace the earlier hospital in 1864–8, with accommodation for 296. It was one of the largest early pavilion-plan hospitals – a block system with detached buildings where a small number of patients are treated in each block.*

Left: *A nurse's uniform was similar to that of a domestic servant. This photograph was taken in the garden of a residential house and the back reads: 'I had this taken at the place I am nursing, love Nellie.' For most of the nineteenth century wealthy people preferred to be treated at home rather than in hospital. Nurses could be hired out privately by the hospitals which had trained them.*

Below: *A postcard of St Thomas's Hospital, London. These buildings were erected in 1868–71 at enormous expense on a site opposite the Houses of Parliament, after the old hospital was demolished to make way for a railway. St Thomas's was by far the largest pavilion-plan general hospital, providing beds for 600 patients. There were six adjacent ward pavilions, with plenty of space between them. Sanitary towers projected from the pavilions at the end near the river. On one side they contained a bathroom and lavatory and on the other a scullery and closets. A ventilated lobby separated the ward from the sanitary facilities to prevent smells, which were believed to harbour disease, from entering the ward. There was ample floor space around each bed to allow room for students and the requirements of clinical teaching.*

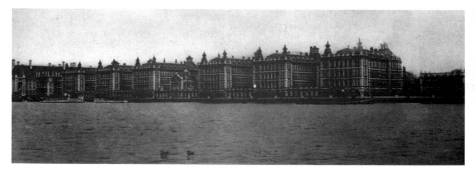

The older hospital design had small rooms leading off a corridor. It was thought that large wards produced disease because of the sheer numbers of sick gathered together in one place. But this did not take into account the difficulty of ventilating small wards and the fact that they also become pestilential when overcrowded. The new pavilion design, widely adopted from the 1860s onwards, had separate ward blocks with plenty of space between them. Another principle of the design was the cross-ventilation of wards by means of pairs of windows opposite each other and two fireplaces to promote the circulation of air to blow away the supposed causes of disease.

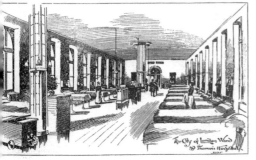

The City of London Ward at St Thomas's Hospital, an accident ward opened in 1899 and typical of the post-Nightingale era. There is a large ward rather than small rooms, with beds placed in two rows, heads against the wall. Although this had the advantage that surveillance by the nursing staff was easy, it took away patient privacy. (Illustration from 'The Hospital', 13th May 1899.)

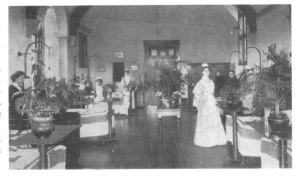

Right: A postcard dated 1909 showing a ward at the Hospital of St Cross, Rugby. The hospital was founded in 1869 but moved to a different location in 1884. The ward was typical for its time: there were plants, parlour palms and flowers; the shiny floor was probably made of oak timber, which was easiest to clean; for the same reason the walls were coated with non-absorbent Parisian cement. On the back wall were polished brass plaques bearing the names of generous benefactors.

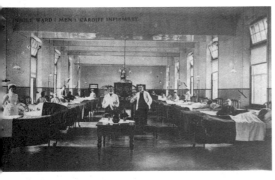

Left: Insole Ward, a men's ward at Cardiff Infirmary, with patients, nurses and (centre) doctors. There were separate wards for men and women, and perhaps for medical and surgical cases, but not for specialisms. Most doctors considered themselves generalists, believing that to specialise was tantamount to admitting to being ill educated. The tall windows are sited opposite each other and are open, to make sure that there is plenty of fresh air. The old theory that ventilation prevented infection remained popular even after the germ theory of disease was accepted. This infirmary was founded in 1822 and closed in 1999.

Hospitals of the early nineteenth century have been called 'gateways to death'. Instruments used on one person's wound were used on the next person. After an operation a patient returned to the wards where he would be surrounded by others with open sores and fevers. The linseed poultices used were a hotbed of infection. A common cause of death after an operation was septicaemia, or blood poisoning. However, the death rate in hospitals is a controversial subject; in civilian hospitals it may not have been as high as is sometimes suggested. In practice, the number of operations attempted was very small because of the high chance of death.

Early-Victorian surgeons had to operate swiftly to minimise pain. Slow, precise or invasive operations were lethal. However, from the 1840s there were important advances in medical science, such as the use of ether and chloroform as anaesthetics. Although anaesthesia reduced the agony of surgery, it did not make it any safer. Even

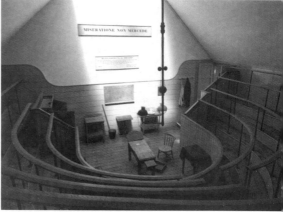

The Old Operating Theatre of Old St Thomas's Hospital, London. This is the oldest surviving operating theatre in Britain. It was built in 1822, before the introduction of anaesthetics and antiseptic surgery.

following Florence Nightingale's advice on ventilation and cleanliness did not totally remove the 'inbred disease of hospitals'.

Another few years passed before Joseph Lister discovered antisepsis. By investigation in the laboratory and hospital wards he proved that the unhealthy condition of septic wounds was due to the action of germs or micro-organisms. Before this, the cause of 'the plague of hospitals' had been a mystery. The practical problem was how to kill the germs without hurting the wound or delaying its healing. In 1865 Lister used carbolic acid for dressing wounds to reduce post-operative infections. As surgery became more feasible surgeons dared to attempt more ambitious operations. More operating theatres were built and they came to be an important part of the hospital. Antiseptic treatment widened the range of surgery as new operations were introduced. Wealthier patients, who traditionally were treated at home, wanted to be admitted too, as they could now get a higher standard of treatment in hospital.

At about this time voluntary hospitals began to provide beds which could be paid for by better-off patients. The effect was to transform hospitals from charities for the sick poor to medical institutions that offered the hope of a cure.

Medical science progressed as doctors learned from observing a large group of patients with the same disease, gathered together in hospital. As their understanding of illnesses improved and they discovered new treatments, doctors began to enjoy high status. Under the Medical Act of 1858 the General Medical Council became responsible for supervising a register of qualified doctors. Doctors started to be appointed by other medical men on the basis of their professional merits. Previously, honorary physicians and surgeons had been elected by the committee of governors of a hospital, which meant that success depended on the candidate's skill at canvassing

Antiseptic dressings and disinfection led to a reduction in hospital diseases. Joseph Lister soaked his surgical instruments in a solution of carbolic acid, used carbolic-soaked dressings and later a carbolic spray to try to kill germs in the air. Carbolic is an unpleasant substance and experiments were made with other antiseptics. Lister also introduced sterile catgut for sutures; it gradually dissolves and is absorbed, so that the stitches do not have to be removed. (Advertisement from 'The Medical Press and Circular', 12th February 1896.)

8

Thermal sterilisation was used to disinfect instruments, dressings and clothing by the 1890s. A small furnace under the machine heated it to produce steam. Hot air was drawn through the machine to dry the articles. (Illustration from 'The Medical Annual', 1896.)

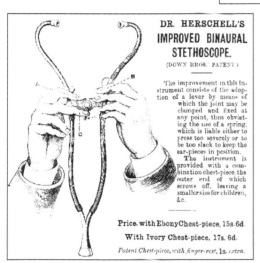

rather than his fitness for the job. Medical students needed bedside experience on the wards, not just anatomy classes, so hospitals became a focus for medical education. By 1900 hospitals had become places in which patients could expect to be cured. Voluntary hospitals had evolved into significant and prestigious centres of research and teaching.

Left: At the start of the nineteenth century a doctor would make a diagnosis based on what the patient told him. Later thorough physical examinations began to be made. A stethoscope was used to diagnose disease. There were many different designs and from the 1850s models with two earpieces were available. The stethoscope was a symbol of the new scientific style of medicine; today it is still recognised as a doctor's 'badge of office'. (Advertisement from 'The Medical Press and Circular', 1896.)

Below: Thermometers had been used for a long time but doctors did not start to use them scientifically to diagnose conditions until febrile diseases were found to have identifiable patterns of temperature variation over time. (Advertisement from 'The Medical Annual', 1896.)

Voluntary hospitals

Voluntary hospitals were philanthropic, charitable institutions initially intended to serve the poor without charge. They were funded from donations and subscriptions. Most were built in the period 1750–1800 and by the mid nineteenth century there were about 250 in Britain. As a town grew, the need for a hospital would become more and more urgent. Typically a group of local worthies would get together to raise funds to establish a hospital for the benefit of the poorer inhabitants of the town. The hospital was governed by a committee of benefactors, which appointed the staff. The buildings were imposing and formal in appearance and included well-appointed reception rooms to accommodate the governors. The impressive buildings were meant as an encouragement to the benefactors and an expression of local pride.

In early Victorian times admission to the hospital was not a decision for one of the doctors: patients needed a letter of recommendation from one of the hospital benefactors. The great and the good liked to give to the voluntary hospitals because the power to admit poorer folk to hospital gave them superior social status in the community. Later, the letter system was dropped because it was an obstacle to the admission of urgent and deserving cases. Instead, patients simply presented themselves at the hospital; a doctor assessed the extent of their medical need and enquiries were made about their financial circumstances.

On arriving at the hospital, or 'The House' as the staff called it, the patient first entered the main hall. Leading off from the main hall was the receiving room, the 'great sieve' of the hospital. All patients had to pass through it before they could be treated, as either an in-patient or an out-patient. It was open day and night, and hundreds of patients would turn up every day. Today, patients are usually referred by their general practitioner to a hospital doctor but in Victorian times hospitals were

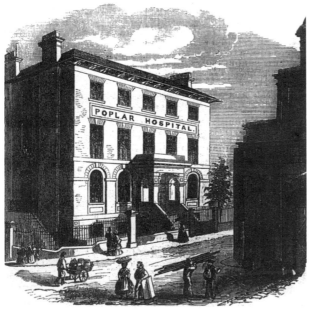

The story of the founding of the charitable Poplar Hospital for Accidents in London is typical. Some philanthropic gentlemen saw that, as more housing and industry developed around London, accidents were happening further and further away from the London Hospital. They held a fund-raising dinner at a hotel, which was attended by many 'highly influential gentlemen'. The hospital also received support from local employers in the area, such as the East India Dock Company. The 'Illustrated London News' noted: 'One of the most satisfactory features is that the working classes give it their support, by weekly subscriptions, annual fêtes, and a variety of performances.' It opened on 1st August 1855 and closed in 1974. (Engraving from the 'Illustrated London News', 12th June 1858.)

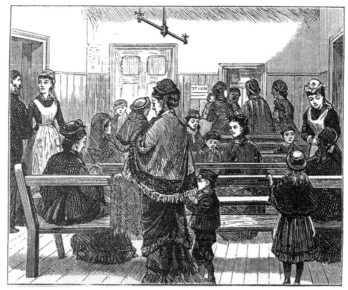

The main hall at the East London Hospital for Children, where patients waited to be seen. Before the GP referral system of today the sick or injured from the poorer classes would go straight to hospital. (Engraving from 'The Graphic', 21st December 1878.)

the first port of call for the sick or injured of the poorer classes. The doctors on duty had to find out quickly whether the patient's condition was minor or serious. If the injury or illness was slight – perhaps a cut finger, a sprain, a sore throat or tooth abscess – the patient was given advice and a supply of medicine or a dressing and sent away. For more serious conditions or those needing a course of treatment, the patient was transferred to the care of the out-patients' department to be thoroughly examined by one of the consultants who visited the hospital. Patients presenting themselves with life-threatening conditions were admitted to one of the wards straight away; only the worst cases could be admitted because there was always a list of patients waiting for a bed to be found.

The hospitals excluded certain kinds of patients on social or medical grounds. The truly destitute were refused, since they were viewed as having moral failings. At the other end of society, patients who could afford to pay for private treatment were also turned away. Incurables, the chronically or mentally ill, and patients with infectious diseases were also barred as nothing could be done for them in hospital. On the other hand, hospitals usually admitted accident cases – a choking child, a man who had fallen down a ship's hold, someone who had been run over, another injured as the result of an explosion, for instance. There were many factory accidents involving unguarded machinery and some employers made special arrangements with the hospital to admit accident cases. As far as the hospital was concerned, the ideal patient was from the respectable labouring poor, and likely to get better soon.

Patients were expected to be extremely grateful for the advice and attention they were given, and some would offer the doctor a tip. Other patients took everything as of right, believing that the hospital was funded from local taxes. One man remarked to a tired and harassed doctor: 'It's the likes of me that keeps the likes of you, and if it wasn't for us being ill, where would you be?' However, hospital doctors were unpaid, their only return being the experience they gained and the hope of making social connections in order to boost their incomes from private business. The doctors' income came from treating wealthier, private patients at home. In the 1840s the upper ranks of society expected to be treated at home, even in surgical cases, rather than to

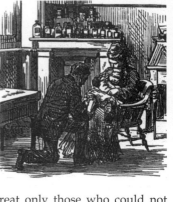

A doctor attending to an accident case. Like all doctors at voluntary hospitals, he would have been an unpaid honorary member of staff. (Engraving from 'The Graphic', 31st March 1877.)

mingle with the masses in hospital. The standard of cleanliness and hygiene was likely to be far higher in a well-off household than in hospital.

Patients sent to the out-patients' department were first seen by an inquiry officer, who determined whether they could receive free medical treatment. They were asked about their earnings, the number of dependent children they had and their rent. This was done out of fairness to the hospital benefactors because the voluntary hospitals were intended to treat only those who could not afford to pay. It was also necessary in order to ensure the doctors' income outside the hospital as private practitioners. The inquiry officer had a difficult job, which necessitated the greatest tact. The dress of patients was never a reliable guide to their means, for many poor people would hire clothes for the day in order to look respectable for their trip to the hospital.

After being passed by the officer, patients waited in the out-patients' waiting hall until called into one of the side rooms to see a house surgeon or physician. By around 1900 hospitals had special equipment for treatments that could not be provided at home. In 1895 X-rays were discovered by Wilhelm Röntgen, and originally called Röntgen rays. Electrical and Röntgen ray departments would be close to the out-patients' department. There, treatment by artificial sunlight – Finsen light – might be used to cure lupus, a disfiguring disease of the skin. X-ray treatment was given for ringworm and tumours. In another room radiographs were taken. Some operators had damaged hands because the danger of X-rays was not known until two or three

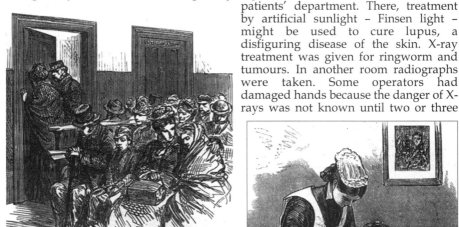

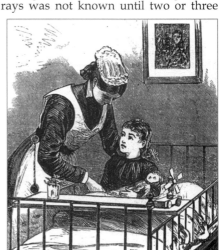

Above: *The out-patients' waiting room at Charing Cross Hospital, London. If a condition needed a course of treatment, the patient became an out-patient and was examined by one of the specialists who visited the hospital. The benches snaked round to form an orderly queue. (Engraving from 'The Graphic', 31st March 1877.)*

Right: *A young patient at the East London Hospital for Children. The iron cots had a sliding table for toys or food that could be pushed towards or away from the child. (Engraving from 'The Graphic', 21st December 1878.)*

12

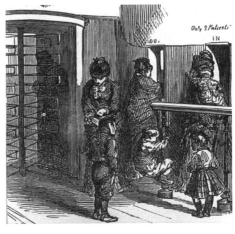

Patients collected their medicine from the dispensing room. Sometimes patients could be seen exchanging sips from their bottles of medicine. The uneducated believed that a medicine which had been good for one patient must be good for all, whatever their ailments! (Engraving from 'The Graphic', 31st March 1877.)

years after their discovery, when those who regularly worked with them started to suffer painful skin inflammation. Later they operated the X-ray equipment from inside a protective lead-lined cabinet, and screens made of glass containing lead were also used.

Sometimes patients were referred to one of the hospital almoners. Many of the cases which arrived at the hospital needed more than strictly medical treatment. The doctor might recommend a diet of meat, cream and milk to build up a convalescent but, for a poverty-stricken patient, he might just as well have prescribed a diet of champagne: it would be impossible to follow the doctor's advice. The almoners were lady volunteers in touch with local charities who could arrange for a patient to be provided with extra food or visited by the local sick-room aid society and health visitors.

Each hospital had an operating theatre; the anaesthetic rooms were separate, so that patients would not see the theatre. The hospital would also have a pharmacy where the medicines were made. After seeing the doctor, patients queued at the dispensary to collect their medicines. Every patient who could afford it paid a few pence towards

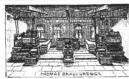
Left: *A hospital would have its own service buildings such as laundry, kitchen, boiler house and mortuary. The Poplar and Stepney Sick Asylum in London had tubes in the walls to convey dirty linen to the laundry, which had washing machines, wringers and mangles worked by steam power, and a large drying closet. (Advertisement from 'The Medical Annual', 1896.)*

Below: *The chapel of the City of London Hospital for Diseases of the Chest. Even the smallest of hospitals had a chapel to cater for the spiritual well-being of the patients. Religion and nursing have a long and close association; senior nurses are called sisters, like nuns. (Engraving from 'The Graphic', 20th March 1886.)*

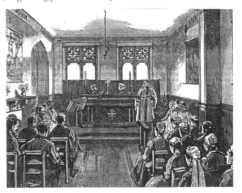

Right: Voluntary hospitals were self-supporting and struggled to attract funds. The traditional ways of raising money were through gala dinners, charity balls and concerts attended by wealthy and prominent supporters. Paying beds were later introduced to raise money and prevent abuse of the charitable work of the institution by better-off patients. The closure of wards due to lack of funds to pay staff was not uncommon. (Advertisement from 'The Hospital', 14th June 1908.)

GREAT NORTHERN CENTRAL HOSPITAL

187 Beds.   17 Beds for Paying Patients.

Holloway, N.

2,300 IN-PATIENTS & 30,000 OUT-PATIENTS ANNUALLY.

NO RESERVE FUND.

£10,000

NEEDED ANNUALLY FROM VOLUNTARY SOURCES.

No Letters Required.   Illustrated booklet describtive of the Hospital and its work post free on application.   Poverty the only Qualification.

L. N. CLENTON-KERR, Secretary.

Below: A street collection for Hospital Saturday. As donations from wealthy benefactors fell relative to costs, hospitals relied more on other forms of fund-raising, such as these appeals. There was also a Hospital Sunday Fund, started in the 1850s, which co-ordinated fund-raising through church collections.

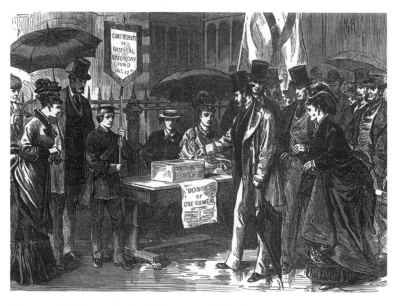

the cost of their medicine. There would also be a kitchen to provide hot meals for the patients, a laundry, a mortuary and a chapel.

By the 1860s medical advances such as the use of anaesthesia and discovery of antisepsis meant that surgeons were able to perform many more operations successfully and wealthier people demanded to be treated in hospitals.

These events coincided with a period of financial difficulty for the voluntary hospitals, which were self-supporting. The donations on which they relied fell relative to costs. Preventing the abuse of charity was a constant headache for the hospital authorities. In response, hospitals introduced paying beds for the richer patients, thereby transforming themselves from charities to medical institutions. Not surprisingly, the paying patients usually had private rooms and a better standard of accommodation. Bed endowment schemes were started and flag days were held in order to raise more money. Working-class people were encouraged to pay into subscription schemes that gave them a right to hospital treatment rather than simply being objects of charity. Many workers gave a penny a week towards the upkeep of the hospital.

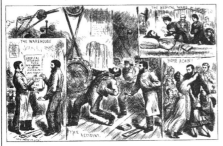

HOSPITAL SATURDAY,
22ND MAY, 1886.

AN APPEAL.

Come and help us, one and all,
Be not deaf to Duty's call ;
Brother toilers pass not by.
Listen to our earnest cry,
   Come, and help us !

Come, O come, with loving heart,
Much or little, do your part ;
Not for us alone the need,
'Tis for you and yours we plead,
   Come, and help us !

Freely give while yet you may,
While in sturdy health to-day ;
Do not linger, do not wait,
Lest to-morrow prove too late,
   Come, and help us !

* * * * *

Swift and sudden falls the blow,
Who the victim none can know ;
You, perchance, who dream no ill,
You, who boast your strength and skill ;
You, as yet, from sorrows free,
You, who still no dangers see ;
Ere the sun shall rise again,
May be faint and worn with pain.

Helpless, hopeless, sad, forlorn,
From your dear ones rudely torn ;
Then, how gladly you would share
Doctor's skill and nurse's care ;
Then, in some bright cheerful ward,
All that science can afford,
All that loving hands can do
Would be freely done for you

* * * * *

Come, then, come without delay,
Join OUR FESTIVAL to-day,
Brother toilers pass not by,
Listen to our earnest cry,
   Come, and help us !

L.B.

Left: *The Hospital Saturday Fund encouraged workers to give a small sum each week (Saturday was usually pay day). Naturally, the workmen who contributed to the fund felt that they had a right to treatment and demand for hospital services increased.*

Below: *The Prince of Wales re-opened Charing Cross Hospital after it had been closed for about a year to allow for alterations and improvements. One ward was named Albert Edward and another Alexandra, after the Prince and Princess. The royal family were important patrons of hospitals, and many hospitals bear the name 'Royal'. One of the most painful cases the Prince and Princess of Wales saw that day was a little child who had had a tracheotomy after swallowing scalding water and lay in an atmosphere continually moistened by steam. (Engraving from 'The Graphic', 31st March 1877.)*

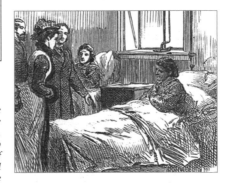

Below: *These stamps, bearing the Prince's signature and a picture of Charity, were issued in 1897 by the Prince of Wales's Hospital Fund, later the King's Fund, to raise money for hospitals in London and as a memento of Queen Victoria's Diamond Jubilee. Even those of limited means could make a small donation. They raised £50,000. The 1898 issue was less successful and the sale of stamps to raise money was abandoned.*

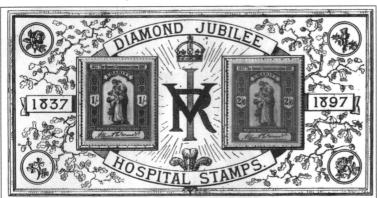

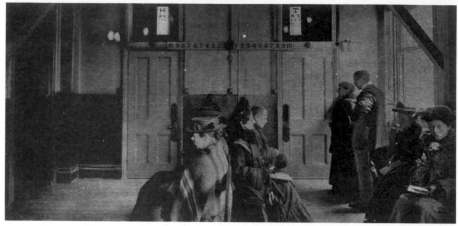

A postcard of the sight-testing room at the Central London Ophthalmic Hospital, founded in 1843. There were several specialist eye hospitals in London. Technical developments such as the invention of the opthalmoscope in 1851 played a part in the expansion of services offered. Sight-testing departments required thoughtful planning as the majority of patients attending were visually impaired. Facilities usually included a waiting-hall, consulting rooms, a minor operations room and a dispensary. Under the National Health Service the Central Hospital became a postgraduate institute within the University of London.

Specialist and cottage hospitals

The general, voluntary hospitals excluded certain categories of patients. As a consequence specialist hospitals were founded, especially from the mid nineteenth century, to deal with neglected groups and the less glamorous areas of medicine.

Sometimes relatives of those who had been touched by a disease started a specialist hospital in order to improve understanding and treatment of the condition. More often entrepreneurial doctors with an interest in a particular condition started their own hospital because they found it difficult to advance their careers within a general hospital. Specialists found that such hospitals gave them the opportunity to study

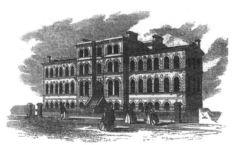

more examples of any single disease than would be found at a general hospital. For this reason admissions to specialist hospitals were decided by doctors rather than benefactors sooner than in the voluntary hospitals. By the 1860s there were sixty-six special hospitals and dispensaries in London alone.

There was a wide variety of specialist hospitals. Some dealt with particular diseases or parts of the body, others with particular age groups. Cancer was rarely

In 1852 Dr William Marsden established a hospital for the treatment of cancer after his wife died of the disease. Originally called the Free Cancer Hospital, it has been known since 1954 as the Royal Marsden Hospital. Facilities did not differ significantly from general hospitals, with large wards on the upper floors and a basement containing a ward for out-patients, with surgeons' rooms and a dispensary, matron's apartments, kitchen and servants' rooms. The discovery at the end of the nineteenth century of X-rays, radioactivity and radium revolutionised the treatment of cancer. Under the National Health Service cancer treatment was gradually integrated into the large general and teaching hospitals. (Engraving from the 'Illustrated London News', 16th August 1862.)

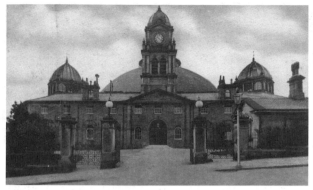

A postcard of Devonshire Hospital, Buxton, Derbyshire. Buxton had a reputation for its healing waters but no proper hospital accommodation was provided until 1858 when the Duke of Devonshire allowed part of his stables and riding school to be converted. The circular exercise yard for the horses was roofed with a wrought-iron dome in 1879 to create an area for the patients' rest and recreation.

treated in general hospitals but was dealt with in specialist institutions. Mineral water and sea-bathing hospitals specialised in arthritis, rheumatism, gout, paralysis and skin complaints. There were eye hospitals and ear, nose and throat hospitals, children's hospitals and hospitals for women. Very few women gave birth in hospital (only about 5 per cent in 1905), but those who did went to a lying-in hospital. There were also orthopaedic hospitals for chronically disabled children, or 'cripples'.

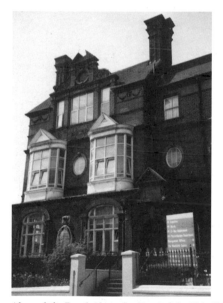

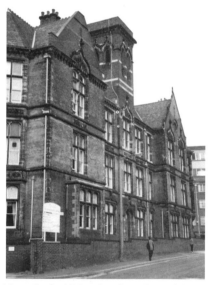

Above left: *Royal Alexandra Hospital for Sick Children, Brighton. In the 1850s, when Great Ormond Street Hospital was founded, children under ten occupied only 3 per cent of hospital beds, although half the deaths in London were of children. The design of children's hospitals was similar to that of general hospitals, as they were essentially general hospitals for little patients. This building dates from 1880.*

Above right: *Jessop Hospital for Women, Sheffield, opened in 1864 to attend cases of midwifery and diseases particular to women. Hospitals for women first appeared in London in the 1840s, as gynaecology emerged as a distinct medical science. The specialist hospitals prompted general hospitals to establish gynaecological facilities. In the twentieth century it was usual to accommodate women's diseases in special departments attached to general hospitals. This picture was taken before the hospital moved to a new building attached to the Hallamshire Hospital in 2001.*

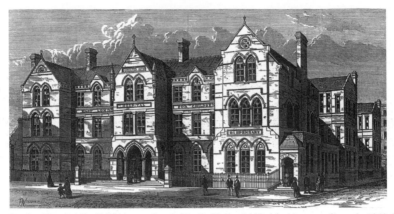

The East London Hospital for Children was founded by Dr Nathaniel Heckford in a warehouse in 1868. It was a dispensary for women too, because a mother's illness could be passed to her child. The new building illustrated here was opened in 1877, when Shadwell High Street was decorated with bunting, and cheering people lined the street. But like all charitable hospitals it struggled to make ends meet. Just a year later 'The Graphic' reported that no more patients could be admitted for want of funds: 'So urgently is money needed, that unless at once forthcoming, this small Ark by the river-side, this small "Star in the East", will before long have practically ceased to exist.' The hospital survived until it was merged in 1942 with the Queen's Hospital for Children in Hackney Road and became one of the group of Queen Elizabeth Hospitals for Children. It finally closed in 1963. (Engraving from the 'Illustrated London News', 12th May 1877.)

Venereal disease was another condition treated in specialist hospitals, sometimes called lock hospitals.

Specialist hospitals caused struggles within the medical profession because in the nineteenth century it was thought that the best doctors were those who were competent in everything. The *British Medical Journal* ran a campaign against specialist hospitals in the 1860s, arguing that they drew away interesting cases from the general hospitals, which harmed the education of medical students. It took a while for specialist hospitals to become respectable, partly because they were a route to personal prestige and wealth for the founding doctor. But specialist hospitals were

A postcard, dated 1905, of the children's ward, Westminster Hospital, London. Hospitals did not at first have separate wards for children; they developed after the establishment of specialist children's hospitals. The atmosphere was formal, with strictly limited visiting hours for parents.

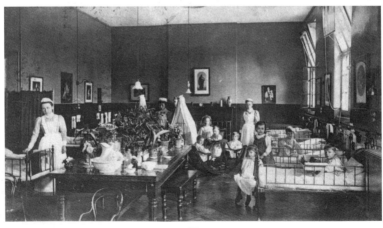

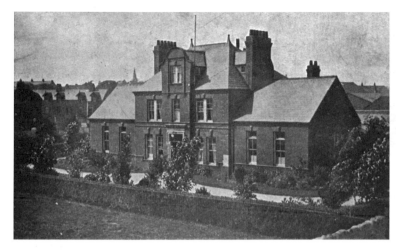

The Queen Victoria Cottage Hospital, Morecambe, Lancashire, founded in 1899. Many 'Victoria Cottage Hospitals' were built to commemorate Queen Victoria's Jubilees.

often responsible for advances in diagnosis and treatment, and by the end of the century the value of taking specialist advice was appreciated more. It became common for a consultant to hold posts simultaneously at a general, voluntary hospital and at a specialist hospital.

Cottage hospitals were established in rural areas from the mid nineteenth century in order to reduce the distances people had to travel for treatment as, hitherto, most voluntary hospitals were concentrated in urban areas, especially London. (Doctors preferred to work in areas where they were more likely to attract large numbers of fee-paying clients.) The patients in cottage hospitals were attended by general practitioners. Having a local hospital advanced the prestige and career of the local doctor, whose patients would otherwise have to go to a large town. Cottage hospitals had between six and twenty-five beds, and they charged a modest weekly sum. In their design cottage hospitals were a world away from most urban hospitals: they had a domestic appearance and were homely, to put patients at ease. The first, archetypal cottage hospital opened at Cranleigh in Surrey in 1859. In 1875 there were 148 cottage hospitals and by 1895 there were nearly 300.

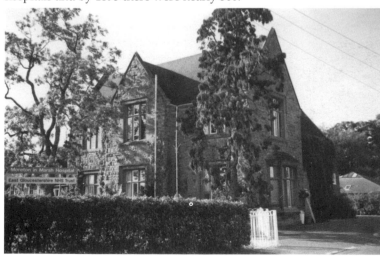

Moreton-in-Marsh District Hospital, Gloucestershire, a former cottage hospital. This view illustrates the domestic appearance which was so characteristic of cottage hospitals.

Poor Law infirmaries

The 1834 Poor Law required people who wanted public relief to enter the workhouse. The legislation made no provisions for the sick; but many inmates were chronically sick or disabled and so a rudimentary hospital service for them gradually developed in the workhouses. In Scotland an Act of 1845 laid down the duty of maintaining proper and sufficient arrangements for the sick poor, including medical attendance. Despite this, the authorities wanted to keep poorhouses as a severe test of genuine poverty, so conditions in the Poor Law hospitals were worse than those in the voluntary hospitals.

Although curable and interesting cases were admitted to the voluntary hospitals, where they were treated by visiting specialist doctors, the aged, infirm or incurable sick ended up at the workhouse hospitals. Workhouse infirmaries lacked out-patients' departments and often operating theatres. Voluntary hospitals depended on workhouse infirmaries as they discharged patients there once the acute stage of illness had passed. Similarly, workhouse infirmaries passed their difficult surgical cases to the voluntary hospitals.

The workhouse hospitals had a grim atmosphere. The functional appearance of the buildings reflected the stigma of the workhouse. In smaller workhouses the buildings were often unsuitable for sick patients. Use as a hospital had not been anticipated in older workhouse buildings. Charles Dickens described 'the foul wards' of Wapping Workhouse: 'They were in a building monstrously behind the time – a mere series of garrets or lofts . . . and only accessible by steep and narrow staircases, infamously ill adapted for the passage upstairs of the sick or downstairs of the dead.' There was hardly any segregation by ailment: 'A-bed in these miserable rooms, here on bedsteads, there on the floor, were women in every stage of distress and disease.'

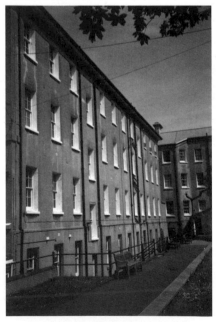

Brighton General Hospital, formerly the town's workhouse and infirmary. This view shows the drab and functional appearance of the workhouse buildings. In contrast, voluntary hospitals had lavish buildings to encourage donations from wealthy benefactors who might become governors of the hospital. The Brighton workhouse was established in 1835 and the infirmary in 1866.

Poor Law doctors were poorly paid, but a quarter of doctors did some Poor Law work, even if part-time. Mill Road Infirmary, Liverpool, was separate from the workhouse buildings, as was increasingly the case after 1867, and was unusual in having a nurse training school. Efforts were made to improve the low standard of nursing in Poor Law infirmaries. One such reformer was Agnes Jones, a pupil of Florence Nightingale, who became matron at Brownlow Hill Institution in Liverpool in 1865. There were 936 probationer nurses in workhouses by 1896 and 2100 by 1901. (Advertisement from 'The Hospital', 17th July 1897.)

The doctors were salaried, unlike the doctors at the voluntary hospitals. The Poor Law created many new posts for doctors but there were difficulties in recruiting practitioners in outlying, poverty-stricken areas where private practice was unremunerative and the prospect of treating mainly chronic and degenerative diseases was unappealing. The medical officer was subordinate to the master of the workhouse and visited once or twice a week. The Boards of Guardians, set up to oversee the running of the workhouses, always wanted to save money and at first the doctor generally had to pay for any medicines out of his own low salary, so the drugs prescribed were limited and alcohol was used frequently.

The daily care of patients was in the hands of the nurses, who were other able-bodied paupers. The standard of nursing was low, but gradually paid, trained nurses were employed instead of the pauper nurses. Louisa Twining was an important crusader for reform. She set up the Association for Promoting Trained Nursing in Workhouse Infirmaries in 1879, but it was difficult to get nurses to work in workhouses where the conditions were relatively poor. In 1897 nursing by pauper inmates was prohibited in England, but this was not practical in Scotland, where there were many small poorhouses that had only an occasional need for nursing and could not justify employing a trained nurse.

A commission to investigate the condition of London's workhouse infirmaries was appointed by the medical journal *The Lancet* and published a critical report in 1865-6. It found fault with the siting, ventilation and sanitation of infirmaries, the lack of segregation of wards, the dependence on pauper nurses and the working conditions of Poor Law medical officers. The Association for Improving London Workhouse Infirmaries was founded in 1866 and the findings of a government inquiry published in the same year broadly agreed with the conclusions of *The Lancet*. The outcome of these initiatives was the Metropolitan Poor Law Amendment Act of 1867, which enabled Poor Law unions in London to establish separate Poor Law infirmaries from

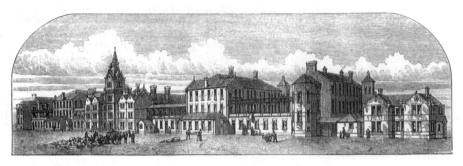

Poplar and Stepney Sick Asylum, East London, built after the 1867 Metropolitan Poor Law Amendment Act, which placed inmates of workhouses who required medical attendance in separate infirmaries. Some new infirmaries, such as this one, were built on separate sites away from the workhouse. A pavilion-plan hospital for 600 patients, it had four separate blocks, two either side of the administrative block. A well-ventilated ground-floor corridor kept the blocks isolated from each other. There was a terrace above this corridor so that convalescent patients could take the air. (Engraving from the 'Illustrated London News', 1871.)

the workhouse. There was no change in the law relating to provincial workhouses, although in 1868 the Poor Law Board recommended that in the larger workhouses the sick should be divided according to the type of case. The majority of Boards of Guardians rebuilt or improved their infirmaries. The new infirmaries all had a separate management from the workhouses, with a resident medical superintendent in charge of medical staff. The principles of pavilion planning started to appear in workhouse infirmaries.

Removing parish patients to the workhouse hospital reduced the distance the Poor Law medical officer had to travel to make visits, so the infirmary ceased to be just for inmates who fell sick and people were increasingly admitted straight into the infirmary. Shortly after the reforms of the 1860s roughly one third of Poor Law infirmary entrants were non-paupers; the 1883 Diseases Prevention Act legalised the admission of non-paupers into Poor Law infirmaries in London. Nevertheless, they remained tainted by association with poor relief. In a few areas the public hospital was of a high standard, but these were the exception. In Scotland, Glasgow led the way in upgrading the hospital part of its poorhouses and providing purpose-built Poor Law hospitals separate from the poorhouses. Bed numbers in the Poor Law sector rose from 50,000 in 1861 to 80,000 in 1911, which was about four times the number provided in the voluntary sector.

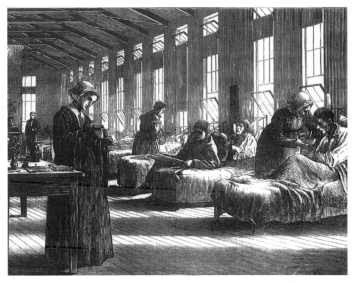

A ward in the Hampstead Smallpox Hospital in London, which was a temporary building of iron and timber huts. At the time it was one of four fever and smallpox hospitals under the management of the Metropolitan Asylums Board in which 24,000 patients were treated during the smallpox epidemic of 1870. Smallpox was the most dreaded illness and there was widespread opposition to the hospital from the residents of Hampstead. The MAB borrowed hulks moored on the bank of the Thames to use as floating hospitals during the epidemics of 1871–2 and 1880–1. (Engraving from the 'Illustrated London News', 7th October 1871.)

Hospitals for infectious diseases

Special hospitals were established to isolate patients with infectious diseases and prevent the spread of infection. Some were public hospitals run by the local authorities and under the control of the local Medical Officer of Health. Others consisted of special accommodation within a workhouse. Their remit was not to relieve individual suffering but to prevent disease. In some areas no charge was made and patients were admitted irrespective of income in order to encourage local inhabitants to enter the hospital, thus protecting the health of the rest of the

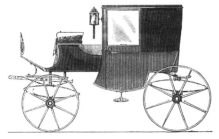

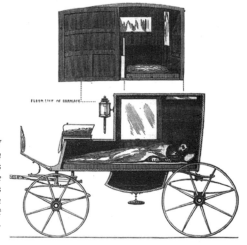

The Metropolitan Poor Law Amendment Act of 1867 set up the Metropolitan Asylums Board to provide a central unified body for treating both infectious diseases and insanity in London. During the next twenty-five years a comprehensive network of fever hospitals was created around London, linked by a horse-drawn ambulance service. The ambulance was designed so it could be thoroughly cleaned to prevent infection. (Engraving from the 'Illustrated London News'.)

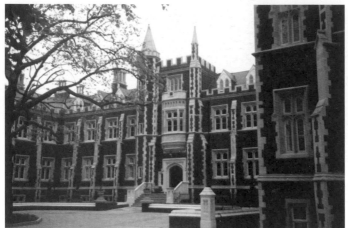

Left: *The Brompton Hospital for Consumption and Diseases of the Chest, London, founded in 1841 by a layman, Philip Rose, who found it impossible to gain admission to any general hospital for one of his employees who had tuberculosis. These buildings were originally designed to maintain a warm, dry atmosphere, thought to be beneficial for patients.*

Right: *The Royal Sea Bathing Infirmary at Margate in Kent was for scrofula, a tuberculosis disease of the glands, joints and bones. The building opened in 1796. Its radical design facilitated the use of sea air and sunshine as part of the treatment for tuberculosis. However, these experiments were contrary to accepted medical opinion of the time.*

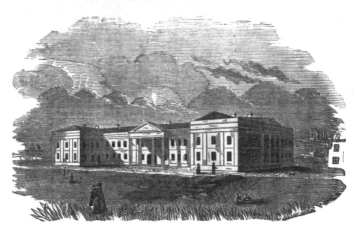

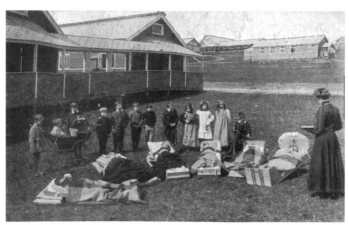

Left: *The Lord Mayor Treloar Hospital, Alton, Hampshire, established in 1908 for the treatment of children suffering from tuberculosis of the limbs and joints. The buildings were originally erected for casualties of the Boer War. Crippled boys learned skilled handicrafts so that they could earn their own living. These children are having their classes in the open air. Some of the children are lying on frames which were used to cure deformities of the limbs and joints caused by TB. The hospital closed in the mid 1990s.*

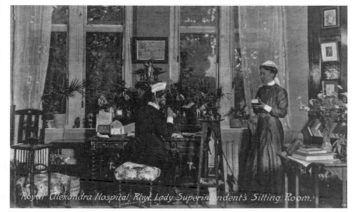

A postcard showing the superintendent's sitting room at the Royal Alexandra Hospital, Rhyl, in North Wales. This institution was founded in 1872 and advocated fresh air as an integral part of the treatment for crippled children. Patients were not discharged until they were cured, even though this process could take years.

population. Still, those who were better off were usually isolated in a separate bedroom at home. Fever hospitals were often temporary structures, erected in response to a local outbreak of smallpox, measles, diphtheria, scarlet fever, or one of the many other serious infectious diseases so prevalent in Victorian times. As a result, few of the old buildings survive today.

Pulmonary tuberculosis was then known as phthisis or consumption. It was identified as infectious only in 1865, but it had long been treated in separate hospitals because it was incurable. In the nineteenth century, treatment of pulmonary TB was limited to boosting the sufferer's immune system. The first private hospitals for consumption tried to do this by creating a dry, warm atmosphere with closed windows, rest and sedation and a limited diet with little or no meat. However, the general acceptance of open-air treatment towards the end of the nineteenth century revolutionised the design of TB hospitals. Verandas, balconies and sun-baths were soon standard features of TB sanatoria.

Mount Vernon Hospital, Northwood, Middlesex. This tuberculosis hospital was built around 1902. The patients are outside taking the fresh air and all the doors and windows are open. A large conservatory where patients could take the sun can also be seen. Once a cure was discovered, TB hospitals were no longer needed but many stayed open because of the special skills of their staff. Mount Vernon Hospital developed a Radium Institute and specialised in cancer. Hospitals for non-pulmonary TB covered in their balconies to provide more beds for the growing speciality of orthopaedics.

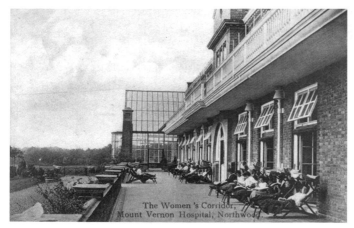

Asylums

The mentally ill were accommodated in lunatic asylums. There were more beds in asylums than in any other kind of hospital in Victorian times. Throughout the nineteenth century the number of certified lunatics steadily increased. More asylums were built and they just kept filling up. Asylum patient numbers rose from 12,000 in 1850 to 27,000 in 1870; by 1900 there were over 100,000 asylum inmates.

Asylums were the first hospitals to be provided from public funds as a result of the 1808 County Asylums Act, which granted permission to build asylums. Before the mid eighteenth century, mental disorder was not recognised as a distinct condition and mentally ill people were generally treated as criminals, paupers or vagrants. For a long time Bethlem Hospital in London was the only charitable hospital for the mentally ill. There were also many private madhouses founded in the eighteenth century, but they were run for profit and conditions in them were deplorable. Garments to restrict the movements of those considered violent were almost universally used until the end of the eighteenth century. Treatments included revolving chairs and cold showers. It was not until the 1830s that attempts were made to reform the county asylums, the lead coming from Hanwell Asylum in London. The idea of non-restraint gradually gained acceptance. Surroundings were improved and patients were encouraged to take part in recreational pursuits, but only a small minority ever left the asylums 'cured'.

Legislation in 1845 made the provision of county asylums compulsory, funded from the local poor rate, and a large number of asylums were built; by 1890 there were sixty-six in England and Wales. To prevent abuses, Lunacy Commissioners were appointed to make regular inspections across the country. A comprehensive network of county asylums developed. They filled up with 'pauper lunatics' whose fees were paid by the local Poor Law Boards of Guardians. For financial reasons, from the 1870s it was the policy to leave harmless cases in the workhouse and send away only the

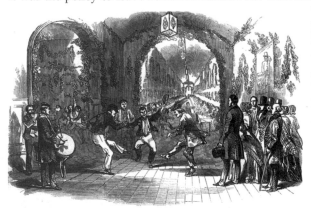

dangerously insane to the asylums. The situation in Scotland was different. The Lunacy (Scotland) Act of 1857 provided for district asylums for the poor throughout Scotland but also allowed harmless lunatics to be boarded in private households, where they were supervised by a regular system of visiting. In London an Act of 1867 created the Metropolitan Asylums Board, which

The first of London's county asylums was Hanwell Asylum, later St Bernard's Hospital. At the time mechanical restraint was considered essential but John Conolly, the medical superintendent of Hanwell, led the way in promoting humane treatment by non-restraint. He maintained that security could be achieved through surveillance by attendants and timely intervention with kind and judicious words. Here the patients are enjoying a dinner and dance and the image is supposed to portray the order and cheerfulness of the institution. By 1860 asylums of 500–800 beds were common. They became 'lunatic colonies' with a largely custodial role, where individual treatment was impossible. Hanwell had more than a thousand beds. (Engraving from the 'Illustrated London News', 15th January 1848.)

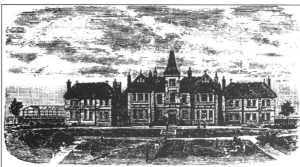

administered hospitals for the insane in the capital.

As well as the county asylums there were also private asylums for paying patients. Scotland had seven voluntary Royal Mental Asylums, which were mainly for private patients. Another well-known hospital was Holloway Sanatorium in Surrey, which provided a well-ordered environment that was considered more suitable for middle-class ladies and gentlemen. The buildings were fine as it was believed that comfortable surroundings would lift the spirits of the patients.

Early asylums typically had long, wide galleries with rows of single cells leading off from them; the galleries doubled as day-rooms for patients. Asylum design evolved to give dormitories and separate recreation rooms, with patients being classed by means of an even wider range of categories, such as quiet or turbulent, chronic or curable. The asylums were often huge, housing hundreds of patients. They were usually isolated outside the town in extensive grounds with an imposing gateway and sweeping gravel drive leading up to the main building. They formed small, self-sufficient communities. Even accommodation for the staff was on site. Work was provided for the patients on the kitchen farm or in the workshops, partly as a form of therapy and partly in order to save money. The main aim was protection of the public. Since the role of asylums was largely custodial, it was more important for the asylum staff to be competent administrators of a gigantic institution than knowledgeable about medical science.

Private philanthropy was responsible for the first asylums specially for people with

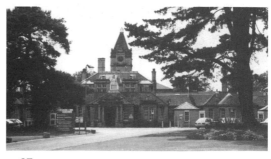

The Warneford Hospital, Oxford, founded in 1826 as a private asylum. Payment was according to a sliding scale. Asylums were often on rural sites near towns to promote tranquillity, to provide outdoor work for patients, and because land was cheaper on the outskirts. These buildings were added in 1877.

Right: *Dr Andrew Reed established a small asylum at Highgate, London, for children with learning disabilities. This led to the erection of the Royal Earlswood Asylum near Redhill in Surrey, opened by Prince Albert in July 1855, with the aim of educating people with learning disabilities, who until then had been widely believed to be ineducable. There was a sense of optimism that they could be trained to become independent. The institution also relieved the family of its financial and caring burden. The original intention was to admit young patients who would stay a maximum of five years, and not beyond the age of fifteen. This aim was not achieved and the trend for large, long-stay institutions was confirmed. (Engraving from the 'Illustrated London News', 31st March 1849.)*

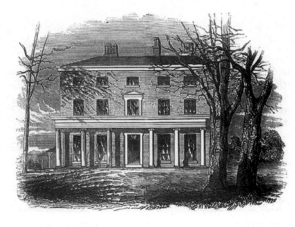

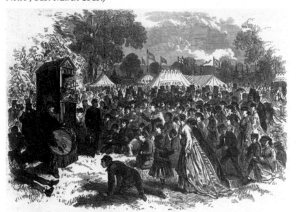

Left: *A summer festival at the Royal Earlswood Asylum, Surrey, to raise funds and entertain the patients. The hospital governors were exclusively male. Nevertheless, women were active in other ways, especially in fund-raising activities and arranging treats for inmates. The newspaper report on the festival noted that: 'a number of useful fancy articles, the productions of the patients, were displayed on stalls, and offered for sale by the ladies of the neighbourhood.' (Engraving from the 'Illustrated London News', 1867.)*

Right: *A hospital election ticket for the Eastern Counties' Asylum for Idiots, Colchester, Essex, established in the 1850s. Subscribers were entitled to vote on the admission of inmates; children were selected if they were the right age and likely to benefit from the regime. A few inmates were funded by Poor Law guardians, but at most asylums the inmates elected were fee-paying. Only a very few children were in special institutions; most people with learning disabilities in institutions were in workhouses, lunatic asylums or prisons.*

learning disabilities. One such institution was the Royal Earlswood Asylum near Redhill in Surrey. These institutions aimed to train the inmates to be independent. There were only a very few special institutions and most 'idiots', as they were called at the time, were looked after in workhouses or county lunatic asylums.

Victorian hospitals today

In 1929 local authorities took over the workhouses, and the Poor Law hospitals were turned into municipal hospitals for the general public, not just the poor. In the 1930s the voluntary hospitals suffered financial difficulties: as scientific knowledge increased, hospital treatments became more and more expensive, and hospitals found it harder to raise enough money to cover their costs from charity collections and subscription schemes.

During the Second World War hospitals came under government control because many civilian casualties from air raids were anticipated. This was the first time that hospital services were unified and centrally directed. This experience paved the way for the creation of the National Health Service. Nearly all hospitals, whether voluntary or municipal, became NHS hospitals in 1948 and hospital treatment became free for everyone regardless of income.

In the early days of the NHS most hospital premises were former Victorian hospitals and workhouses. However, by the second half of the twentieth century many of the old buildings were either no longer needed or considered unsuitable for use as hospitals. The medical profession felt that specialist hospitals should be superseded by special departments within general hospitals, so many of the old specialist institutions were merged with other hospitals. The introduction of antibiotics in the 1940s provided a new, effective treatment for infectious diseases, including tuberculosis, which resulted in a decline in the need for isolation hospitals and TB sanatoria; many were put to new uses or abandoned altogether. In mental health care, drug treatments have improved and the trend has been towards care in the community and wards in general hospitals, so the large, remote asylums are becoming redundant.

Many small hospitals evolved in Victorian times in response to parochial allegiance and charitable initiatives and they were not always situated in the places of greatest need. As hospitals need more and more hi-tech equipment and specialist staff on duty round the clock, larger hospitals have come to be regarded as more efficient. Finding the best way to re-organise hospital services has not been easy, and the closure of

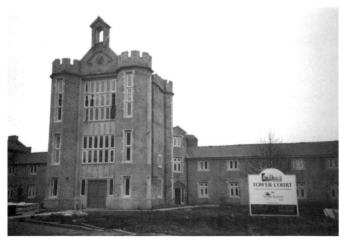

Tower Hospital, Ely, Cambridgeshire, undergoing conversion to luxury flats in 2000. This former workhouse and Poor Law infirmary was founded in 1837 and closed in 1993. Many Victorian hospitals have been sold off for redevelopment.

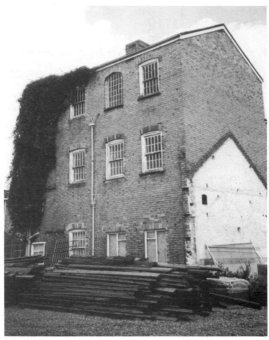

The infirmary block of the former Chesterton Union workhouse, Cambridge, originally erected in 1836–8. The sexes were separated, with two men's wards on the top floor, a lying-in ward and a women's ward on the first floor, and a surgeon's room and storeroom on the ground floor. It later became Chesterton Hospital but by 2000, when this photograph was taken, most of the site was no longer in use and demolition work was taking place.

some hospitals has been met with fierce local opposition. Yet gradually Victorian hospitals are closing and being sold off for redevelopment. Some have become luxury apartments; others are used as residential homes for the elderly.

What role did Victorian hospitals play in improving the health of the people? On one hand this is a difficult question to answer as there are few sources of historical evidence on the extent of illness. On the other hand, historians know a great deal about when people died. Life expectancy at birth rose in England and Wales from just over age forty-five in the 1830s to sixty-eight in 1911, and a simultaneous reduction in illness is generally assumed to have occurred. But most historians agree that advances in medical treatment did little to improve the health of the mass of the population. Poor diet, dangers in the workplace, overcrowded housing, the incidence of infectious diseases and pollution of the environment were all more important influences. The real advances in health in Victorian times were due to improvements in nutrition and public health made possible by engineering, not medicine. Nevertheless, in the course of the age, the small number of institutions serving a minority of the population grew into the network of hospitals still familiar to us today, with the prospect of a cure becoming surer as knowledge increased.

Further reading

Abel-Smith, Brian, and Pinker, Robert. *The Hospitals, 1800–1948: A Study in Social Administration in England and Wales*. Heinemann, 1964.

Bynum, W. F. *Science and the Practice of Medicine in the Nineteenth Century*. Cambridge University Press, 1994.

Cherry, Steven. *Medical Services and the Hospitals in Britain, 1860–1939*. Cambridge University Press, 1996.

Emrys-Roberts, Meyrick. *The Cottage Hospitals, 1859–1990*. Tern, 1991.

Gale, Colin, and Howard, Robert. *Presumed Curable: An Illustrated Casebook of Victorian Psychiatric Patients in Bethlem Hospital*. Wrightson Biomedical Publishing, 2003.

Jones, Kathleen. *Asylums and After: A Revised History of the Mental Health Services*. Athlone, 1993.

Lane, Joan. *A Social History of Medicine: Health, Healing and Disease in England 1750–1950*. Routledge, 2001.

O'Neill, Cynthia. *A Picture of Health: Hospitals and Nursing on Old Picture Postcards*. Meadow Books, 1990.

Peterson, M. Jeanne. *The Medical Profession in Mid-Victorian London*. University of California Press, 1978.

Pickstone, John V. *Medicine and Industrial Society: A History of Hospital Development in Manchester and Its Region, 1752–1946*. Manchester University Press, 1985.

Porter, Roy. *Blood and Guts: A Short History of Medicine*. Penguin Books, 2003.

Porter, Roy. *Madness: A Brief History*. Oxford University Press, 2003.

Poynter, F. N. L. (editor). *The Evolution of Hospitals in Britain*. Pitman Medical Publishing Company, 1964.

Richardson, Harriet (editor). *English Hospitals 1660–1948: A Survey of Their Architecture and Design*. Royal Commission on the Historical Monuments of England, 1998.

Rivett, G. *The Development of the London Hospital System, 1823–1982*. King Edward's Hospital Fund for London, 1986.

Waddington, Keir. *Charity and the London Hospitals, 1850–1898*. Royal Historical Society, 2000.

Woodward, John. *To Do the Sick No Harm: A Study of the British Voluntary Hospital System to 1875*. Routledge & Kegan Paul, 1974.

The histories of many individual hospitals have been published, although they may be out of print. Local studies centres or libraries are good places to look for such books.

The Hospital Records Database, a joint project of the Wellcome Trust and the Public Record Office, provides information on the existence and location of the records of hospitals in the United Kingdom. It is available on-line: http://hospitalrecords.pro.gov.uk/

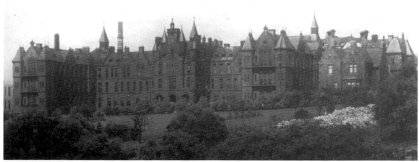

A postcard of the Western Infirmary, Glasgow. Universities and hospital medical schools became the centres for the clinical instruction of medical students in the nineteenth century. The Western Infirmary opened in 1874 with 200 in-patient beds to provide a teaching hospital adjacent to the university's new site at Gilmorehill. Before that students had to travel to the older Glasgow Royal Infirmary.

Places to visit

There are many Victorian hospitals still standing in Britain – most towns have one. Some are no longer suitable for use as hospitals and have been turned into old people's homes, office buildings, housing developments and even hotels.

A list of hospital sites is contained in the back of *English Hospitals 1660–1948: A Survey of Their Architecture and Design*, edited by Harriet Richardson. Files containing research and photographs created by the Royal Commission on the Historical Monuments of England are available at the National Monuments Record Centre, Kemble Drive, Swindon SN2 2GZ. Telephone: 01793 414600.

The following is a list of places where you can learn more about the history of hospitals and medicine. Readers are advised to telephone to find out opening times and days.

Bethlem Royal Hospital Archives and Museum, Monks Orchard Road, Beckenham, Kent BR3 3BX. Telephone: 020 8776 4227. Website: www.bethlemheritage.org.uk A collection of works of art by artists who experienced mental disorder and other material from the seventeenth century to the nineteenth century relating to the history of psychiatry.

Crichton Museum, Crichton Royal Hospital, Dumfries. Telephone: 01387 244000 or 244228. Situated in the grounds of Crichton Royal Hospital, this museum is devoted to the story of mental health care during the last 200 years and has a collection of art work by patients going back to Victorian times.

Florence Nightingale Museum, St Thomas's Hospital, 2 Lambeth Palace Road, London SE1 7EW. Telephone: 020 7620 0374. Website: www.florence-nightingale.co.uk Presents the life of Florence Nightingale, her work in the Crimea and her creation of the first modern nurse training school.

George Eliot Hospital Museum, 4th Floor Maternity Hospital, George Eliot Hospital NHS Trust, College Street, Nuneaton, Warwickshire CV10 7DJ. Telephone: 024 7686 5540. Website: www.geh.nhs.uk/Depts/Museum/home.htm Medical artefacts from the nineteenth and twentieth centuries are on display in this museum.

George Marshall Medical Museum, Charles Hastings Education Centre, Worcestershire Royal Hospital, Charles Hastings Way, Worcester WR5 1DD. Telephone: 01905 760738. The museum leads the visitor through the history of medicine with room settings and interactive displays. The exhibits include an early-nineteenth-century operating theatre.

Glenside Hospital Museum, Faculty of Health, University of the West of England, Blackberry Hill, Stapleton, Bristol BS16 1DD. Telephone: 0117 965 2688. Artefacts from the history of psychiatry and people with learning difficulties are on display in the chapel of this former county asylum built in 1861.

Leicester Royal Infirmary History Museum, Knighton Street Nurses' Home, Royal Infirmary, Leicester LE1 5WW. Telephone: 01858 565532. Website: www.uhl-tr.nhs.uk Tells the story of the infirmary, founded in 1771.

Museum of the Royal College of Surgeons of England, 35–43 Lincoln's Inn Fields, London WC2A 3PE. Telephone: 020 7869 6560. Website: www.rcseng.ac.uk This museum is due to re-open in early 2005 following a major refurbishment.

Old Laundry Medical Museum, Royal Berkshire Hospital, Reading. Postal address: Berkshire Medical Heritage Centre, Level 4 Main Entrance, Royal Berkshire Hospital, Reading, Berkshire RG1 5AN. Telephone: 0118 926 2724. Website: www.bmhc.org Has medical, surgical, nursing, pharmacy and dental equipment, documents and photographs mainly from the Victorian period to the mid twentieth century.

The Old Operating Theatre, Museum and Herb Garret, 9a St Thomas Street, London SE1 9RY. Telephone: 020 7955 4791. Website: www.thegarret.org.uk A pre-anaesthetic operating theatre with a nineteenth-century wooden operating table and observation stands. The museum displays the history of herbal medicine, Old St Thomas's, Guy's and Evelina Children's Hospitals, and Florence Nightingale's nursing school.

Royal London Hospital Archives and Museum, St Augustine with St Philip's Church, Newark Street, Whitechapel, London E1 2AA. Telephone: 020 7377 7608. Website: www.brlcf.org.uk The London, founded in 1740, became Britain's largest voluntary hospital; museum includes nursing uniforms, equipment and surgical instruments.

St Bartholomew's Hospital Museum and Archives, St Bartholomew's Hospital, West Smithfield, London EC1A 7BE. Telephone: 020 7601 8152. Website: www.brlcf.org.uk Tells the story of one of the oldest hospitals in the world.

The Science Museum, Exhibition Road, South Kensington, London SW7 2DD. Telephone: 0870 870 4868. Website: www.nmsi.ac.uk Exhibits related to the history of medicine.

Stephen G. Beaumont Museum, Field Head Hospital, Ouchthorpe Lane, Wakefield, West Yorkshire WF1 3SP. Telephone: 01924 328654. Depicts the history of the Stanley Royd Hospital, a former pauper lunatic asylum founded in 1818.

Thackray Medical Museum, Beckett Street, Leeds LS9 7LN. Information hotline: 0113 245 7084. Telephone: 0113 244 4343. Website: www.thackraymuseum.org Traces the history of medicine from the ordeal of surgery before anaesthetics to the discovery of modern medicines.

The website www.medicalheritage.co.uk lists museums, libraries and other sites of medical interest around Britain.

The website www.medicalmuseums.org has information about London's museums of health and medicine.